Beyond The Combs

A Celebrity Hairstylist's Guide to Success

By Rhonda O'Neal

TO GOD BE THE GLORY!

To my wonderful, amazing mother, Barbara Stroman (Mrs. B) thank you for igniting the spark under me and teaching me all that I know.
To my amazing dad, Eugene Stroman Sr. for holding The Hair Masters down as my receptionist.
I just have to say without the two of you I would be nothing. From a daughter that will always cherish and never take lightly the love of her parents. I know the two of you have been watching over me every step of my journey called LIFE. I will always love you and miss you both. To my wonderful siblings Karen, Eugene Jr., and Nicole, without our own journeys we wouldn't be where we are today. I love you.

And to the Bright lights that always keep me in the straight tunnel even when they don't want to Terry II., Te'Rhon, and Tyra; my amazing children. Thank you for your patience and being there every step of the way. I love all of you.

CONTENTS

Introduction

Celebrity Hairstylist's Guide To Success

THANK YOU

Shondrella Avery

Shaun Robinson

Judge Mablean Ephrian

Eric Andre

Andre Braugher

Kevin Frazier

Kenneth Walker

Italy Hair Products

Frends Beauty Suppy

Nigel's Emporium

Wen Products by Chaz

Hair and Makeup Artist Network, www.hmartistsnetwork.com

Front cover credits:
Photo by
Regi kim
vmecommunications@gmail.com

Makeup by Jerry Kimbell
jerrykimbell@yahoo.com

Back cover credits:
Photo by
www.ericscot.com

Makeup by
Dionne Wynn
makeupbydionnewynn@gmail.com

INTRODUCTION

"ENTREPRENEURSHIP…is living a few years of your life like most people won't, so that you can spend the rest of your life like most people can't." - unknown

When I decided to write this book I knew there were thousands of books on the market today, but I also knew it would be different because my experiences were different. My journey has been different from someone else's journey. For that reason, I pushed forward and I wanted to share it with you. I'm hoping as you're reading this book it will help you on your journey to teach and inspire you to challenge and overcome your limitations while at the same time strive to fulfill your highest possible purpose as one of the best creative artists to ever walk this earth.

In doing so I want to make sure I gain a personal relationship with you through my writings. My goal is to inspire and provide you with the necessary tools and practical guidance to help you breakthrough whatever's stopping you from reaching your highest potential life has to offer. Knowing from experience through hard work and determination many rewards await you. With that being said I don't know that 365 days from today your life will be better or worse, but what I do know is that it won't be the same. No matter where each one of us starts out on the socioeconomic scale we all have the potential for greatness. I want to encourage you to stay focus and refuse to accept limitations, either those coming from others or those you place on yourself.

In the title of this book and throughout its pages, I encourage you to rise above any challenges that may come your way, because they ARE going to come. Learn from your mistakes. Build from all of the goodness that you receive and continuously make adjustments so that you will keep your focus to succeed beyond the combs!

I want you to feel each experience that I've encountered. I want you to know this isn't just a book you're reading but it's a relationship being built between us. To me every person I meet is special no matter if they're filthy rich or a person with a heart filled with kindness. It doesn't matter to me who you are but what's important to me is building a relationship with you. I remember my parents saying to me growing up, "Love everybody no matter what their color is, how much money they have, what size they are or what they look like". That has stuck with me all of my life and now that I have the opportunity to bring you into my life through these pages I have just established one more relationship. My sincere hope is to be that guide for you using what my parents instilled in me as light to ignite the fire within you.

Before you get too comfortable. Get up grab yourself a cup of tea, now relax and let's begin this journey together.

Building your success beyond the combs, takes you far beyond styling hair behind the chair in the salon. If you're a makeup artist, it will take you far beyond that makeup counter in the store or even selling Mary Kay to all your girlfriends and relatives. There are other great opportunities as an artist that are available to you, but finding your way is where I come in. I'm going to take you far beyond the combs.

Whatever city or town you live in, believe me you can find ways to do hair or makeup in places other than behind the chair or over the counter. Be the artist that you are and think creatively. There are politicians, churches, businesses, companies and at least 1 radio and/or television station in your hometown. These people want to always look their best in public and they can't always maintain it themselves. They need help. They need YOUR help.

Back when I lived in Missouri City, a suburb of Houston, Texas in the 80's, as a 21 year old salon owner no one would have told me I would be doing hair on major television shows or blockbuster films or on some of the most well-respected actors in Hollywood. But what I did know was that I was a ball of energy just trying to think of the next thing to do to put my salon, The Hair Masters on the map.

My mother, Barbara Stroman (aka Mrs. B), was also a hairstylist and if it weren't for her I know I wouldn't be where I am today. She helped to put me on the path of becoming a hairstylist because my mind was telling me I wanted to go to college and become an architect. My path changed after I managed her salon once I graduated from high school. I fell in love with hair and the rest is history.

But back to the story. I went down to one of the local television stations to see about them advertising my salon but instead I thought maybe I'll ask if I could do the news reporter's hair and they let me because there was no one doing her hair. DING...here's your chance to ask your local station. I did her hair for about a year but it was taking me away from the salon too much so I had to give that job to someone else. Lesson #1: Don't be afraid to spread the wealth. I'm known for referring others to jobs. If you hear of a job that you can't do because you're too busy or you can't perform the task don't think that productions won't ever call you back. One of my mottos is, "If you keep your hand so closed there's nothing else that can go in it".

When you don't share you don't receive more. My life was a whirlwind so I recommended another young lady to take my place. From working there, the people at the station started referring clients to my salon. So, wouldn't one say from me sharing helped me not only to receive more clients but my operators in my salon also benefited. Kindness goes along way. Remember, that was my first goal to put The Hair Masters on the map and it was now happening.

Having the experience of working with a high-profiler was now on my resume. Not realizing how much this would help me 20 years later. I began looking into the local pageants in my city. I started doing hair for the Miss Black Houston Pageant and later the Miss Texas Pageant. People started recognizing my name. Now, I'm doing hair for cable shows and special events. I started being referred to the Houston Rockets, the Oilers at the time and their wives. Believe me, now The Hair Masters was definitely on the map. I had no idea that all that I was doing to get The Hair Masters on the map would benefit me 20 years later. All the different jobs from the newsroom at the television station to styling for pageants to having sports figures and their wives as my clients, was in itself its own entertainment world. I guess you could call it a small town production.

1 DON'T RUSH

"The important thing is to take your time and not get stressed." – Diane Von Furstenberg

Okay, so you're a hairstylist, makeup artist or wardrobe stylist. In the world of entertainment there's not much difference. The steps for being successful in anyone of these areas are basically the same. What you do have to start is creating a plan. If working with magazines and high profile photographers or working on non-union productions to work toward becoming a union hairstylist or makeup artist or stylist is your goal than you have to start implementing it. Whatever your plan is, I will help show you the way.

Your ultimate goal of being a celebrity stylist is going to happen as long as you exercise patience and put the work in. However, I admonish you not to rush the process. This will cause you to skip some very necessary steps. You have to lay the proper foundation in order to achieve the results that you want. You want to make sure that you're at the top of your game before you go for your goal. Olympic athletes train hard before they reach the Olympics. You don't hear about the years of hard work that they've put in, the sleep that they've missed, or the sacrifices. We usually only get to see them at the top of their game, but the truth is that a lot of blood sweat and tears have occurred before they got there. The process to become an Olympian is a long one and it's uncertain. The process is different depending on which sport they play but there are some very basic things that take place in each category.

First, they have to choose a sport and enroll under the instruction of a qualified coach. Then when the coach feels that they're ready, they begin competing in local events; if they're successful in these, they work their way up to state, regional and national competitions. If they achieve a high level of success in the process, it earns them an opportunity to try out for a spot in the Olympics. Each sport has its own national governing board. The governing board is responsible for selecting who gets a chance at being part of an Olympic team and each board has different criteria that they must meet if they want to be considered for a spot on the team. Those who compete in individual sports will likely be able to compete for a spot based on their national rankings and athletes in team sports are generally chosen by a national coaching squad based on their reputation and rankings. There are also a few sport's teams that have Olympic tryouts.

If the board thinks that they will be a valuable addition to the Olympic team then they will be invited to attend the official Olympic team training camp. That is where they are evaluated and ranked. If they finish in one of the top five spots for their sport then they have a good chance in being selected to join the team but the standards vary across the spectrum. After completing the training camp, their fate is in the hands of their sport's Olympic coach. The coach has the final say on which athletes will representing the USA in the next Olympic games.

You may be wondering why I took you through the entire process of becoming an Olympian. I did it because it's how I see the industry. There are so many steps that you have to go through in order to become a celebrity stylist and they're all important. You can't skip anything. It's not realistic to show up at the Olympic camp unprepared and without the proper training or clearances and think that you're going to get in. You can't expect to just pop up at a movie set and think that you're going to do someone's hair. Consider me as your coach. Allow me to teach you how to get into the celebrity arena. With this guide, you'll have a realistic and uplifting perspective on how to become the celebrity stylist that you've always dreamed of. I'll also be deconstructing some of your beliefs about what the industry is like. It's not as glamorous as some people believe but it is lucrative and it can be very rewarding if you're in it for the right reasons it can be so much fun. So don't rush the process. Do everything that you can right now to become the best hairstylist that you can possibly be and then work from there..

2 WELCOME TO HOLLYWOOD

"I hated every minute of training, but I said, "Don't quit. Suffer now and live the rest of your life as a champion." - Muhammad Ali

Once I moved to Los Angeles I knew I wanted to be my own boss again and so after a couple of failed businesses I pursued my passion again…HAIR. This time things were different. I wasn't a salon owner in my hometown anymore. I had to figure out LA's way of doing hair. Yes, I knew how to do hair and do it well but that was from Texas standards. The trends were different, the weather was different, and the people were definitely different.

As a hairstylist you probably already know how challenging it can be to get into a high end hair salon. Now imagine that times 10 because you're in LA. I had a general idea of how to do this when I moved from Houston to LA and it worked. See, I already had a salon in Houston for almost ten years. Before that, my mom had a salon and it was booming. So high-end clients weren't new to me.

Keep in mind that the terrain in the industry has changed. These are my experiences in L.A., and now they can be yours regardless of where you live. Productions are taking place all over the U.S. So you don't have to move to LA to have the Hollywood experience but now just imagine your town as "Hollywood" and with that comes a change in the way you have to think about your craft. You may have to make a few changes whether that's in moving to a new salon, taking more classes or assisting some of the best stylists in your area.

I've done the hair of entertainers, athletes, doctors and lawyers, their wives etc. When I moved to Los Angeles, I said, "You know, I want to have that same kind of energy around me." And I knew that the only place that I could probably get it would be in another high-end salon. So I went into Beverly Hills, and talked to a couple of people and they told me about a couple of salons and I thought about it, I realized that I didn't know L.A's way of doing hair, so I needed to assist someone. Keep in mind you're having to learn Hollywood's way of doing hair. More fashion forward. #trendy One thing that I'm asked a lot by hairstylists is "How do I find the person that I want to assist, and how do I approach them?" Try working with working hairstylists that have a top notch clientele because you will learn a wealth of information. The best way to go into any situation is with the attitude of, "I'm just here to help."

Ask around to find out who's working with the best of the best and when you approach that person you should have your stuff in order. Make sure your resume is on point when you hand it to them. Even if you've just finished beauty school make sure you show that person how organized and professional you are and can be. Your first impression is lasting.

Someone told me to go meet a guy by the name of Victor Moore, he was a great hairstylist but he had a reputation of having very high standards. He was very particular. This man could walk into an interview and sketch styles that he had in mind for a video or movie. He didn't have to bring photos, he would sketch anything in a matter of seconds. You had to be ready for Victor! He wasn't ordinary he was extraordinary. So needless to say, I was intimidated when I first went into the salon to meet him, but once I did, he was like a little teddy bear. Nice guy, very focused on the world of hair. I knew I was one of the best hairstylist in my hometown so I only wanted to assist one of the best hairstylist in LA. He did so many of the young Who's Who of Hollywood from Holly Robinson Peete to EnVogue. He was damn good. I began working with Victor in the mid '90s when the flat iron craze was just starting. At the time many other cities were not flat ironing. By assisting Victor he taught me LA's way of doing hair. He would teach me LA's way and I would teach him Texas' way.

I did more listening than talking. Even though, I had more years in the business I knew he was someone I could learn from. He was teaching me new things. He was teaching me a new way of looking at hair and the entire hair industry. The more I listened, the more I learned.

Let's be real, I was new to L.A. but I wasn't new to hair. I had over 15 years of experience under my belt. Many hairstylists that have put time into their career would not want to approach their next move this way. Technically, it's a downgrade.

Hairstylist would come to him and ask to be his assistant. Remember in order to grow you have to be willing to step back and learn more. Be an excellent assistant, and learn from a pro. If you decide to be an assistant one piece of advice is to stay in your place as an assistant and as you grow, good things will come to you. Who really wants to assist another hairstylist when they already know what they're doing. I did, and I'll tell you why. Honestly, it saved me in the long run. I had a lot of experience but I didn't have experience in L.A. I realized long ago that being the best hairstylist is not just how well you do hair, it's how well you know people. I knew that the market was different and it would have been naïve for me to think that I would get a high-end clientele without knowing what they wanted and knowing what type of people I was dealing with. These weren't Southern people. Now I lived in a melting pot. So many ethnicities and many different personalities with many different types of hair textures. The way hair is worn in New Jersey is different from the way hair is worn in Chicago. Texas hair is different than L.A Hair.

I knew that in order for me to go from being a good stylist to a great stylist in L.A. I had to work with the best. Victor worked with so many celebrities I can't name them all. I took that time to assist him, learn how to do hair the L.A. way, and it was priceless.

Unfortunately it was short-lived, because he passed away a year and a half later. But I will forever be grateful to him, and I miss him. Thank you Victor for sharing.

My number one piece of advice to those that are trying to make it in L.A. is to be on your A-Game wherever you come from first. Be the one that made it happen in your hometown. Don't think that you're going to come to L.A. and be the "Hairstylist to the Stars" if you didn't put in work in your hometown first. #crushingit There is a lot of work involved to get to that level. I'm not saying that it never happens; I'm saying that it takes time, patience and lots of grinding. Whether it's for free or for pay. You're going to pay lots of dues but in the end it's all worth it. Once you come to L.A. you will have to know how to market yourself, and adjust yourself to whatever is needed. I wasn't from L.A. but I'd already established myself in Houston. Even with my years of experience, I didn't get to start at the top. I still had dues to pay.

When you come into Hollywood, it can be overwhelming. All of the hairstylists are the best of the best. Celebrities are looking for the people at the top of their game. In order to have celebrities as clients, you have to feel comfortable with them. You have to have successfully dealt with a lot of different personalities from a lot of different walks of life. So don't come to Hollywood acting "Hollywood." You're not the star. Keep in mind you want to work with stars. #celebrities

This goes for whatever city or state you're in. Stay humble at all times and remember that it's not about you when you're in the salon, on set, in trailers or even at a photo shoot. I say all the time we're not in the beauty industry, we're in the catering industry. We must know how to cater to others. I call it giving back. #selfless The more you give the more you receive. I guarantee you your blessings will come back to you in some form or another. Sometimes it doesn't come back like you think it should but believe me good will come back to you. As long as your intentions are good.

If now you feel you're ready to be a part of the big league, then do your research. Find out where others like you hangout. Join, The Hair and Makeup Artist Network, www.hmartistsnetwork.com. You can start by talking to different kinds of stylists. From freelancers to union to non-union stylists. Find out their journeys and that can help you get to where you're trying to go. Go into different salons and once you do that, you can get a feel of where you would like to be. When you go into the salons, have a resume of what you've done, state where you're from, and ask if they need an assistant. Cushion yourself, make sure that you are financially stable before you make this move in your career because some assistants will have to work for free. You will basically work off of tips, so a nest egg of money you saved or your parents gave you will make all the difference in how you can obtain your goal. LA is not the place to play around. It can be hard if you don't come here with a thought out plan and once you're here you can build off that plan. I also recommend getting a roommate. Accept the fact that you can't always make it on your own. It takes time. If it happens sooner than later for you, kudos! I grasped as much information as I could while working as an assistant. My motto I tell people is "To always be a student, always be willing to learn more". Ask questions. Because when you're a student, you can rise to the top. You have to remain teachable throughout your career. How else are you going to stay on top of new trends and techniques? Being a student humbles you. Humble people tend to work the most. People are attracted to humbleness.

As I worked with Victor, we became a great team. I had no issues with him being ten years younger than me, for me that was the best thing for me. He lit a spark under me because what I was learning from him was invaluable. I was able to go ten years back in time. I had no problems with saying, "I don't know this or that." Asking questions is the key element when you're dealing with a high profile artist. Stay in your place and don't try to outshine them. Don't be that person that knows it all, because you'll miss out on a ton of great opportunities.

You're studying under them for a reason. Learn why they're in the position that they're in. Being teachable is a key element. You always have to be open to learning because there are always going to be things that you don't know. The industry is always coming up with something new, and there are some older techniques that still work and then they're new ones that are being implemented all the time. Also, you never know where or who this knowledge is going to come from. Don't make assumptions based off of a person's age or experience. Anyone can be filled with valuable knowledge.

3 BEAUTY

"I believe that all women are pretty without makeup and can be pretty powerful with the right makeup." – Bobbi Brown

I remember growing up, one thing my mom would always tell her daughters was, "Don't leave the house without lipstick on". She meant always leave the house looking your best. Beauty is important even more so today than ever. Everywhere you turn now pictures are being taken for social media. Do people judge us by our appearance? ABSOLUTELY! Having a complete look, the whole package from head to toe, your hairstyle, your makeup and what you're wearing is so important these days. That's why the creative artists that we are will always be important to society. Think about it. We spend well over $5 billion a year on hair products and services.

In the creative world I must say our presence is felt on every level. We have beauty and makeup schools, beauty supply stores, beauty salons and now television shows about our creative world. From Tyra Banks' "Top Model" to "Rip the Runway" to "LA HAIR", the beauty world should be more powerful amongst us economically. Many people say I should rest on my laurels now since I've done the owning the salon thing, displayed my artistry in pageants, taught in community colleges, and created styles for movie stars and have worked on blockbuster films and television shows. All the accolades could go to one's head. Instead, they have moved me to a higher level of creative consciousness. I want to be here to help guide you on your road to becoming your best self now. I've learned that just a little tweaking or making a few minor adjustments to your life makes a huge difference. If that means becoming a "Stylist to the Stars" then let's do it. I guarantee you as you take this journey to becoming the best artist you can be you will have fun doing it and on top of that it can be financially rewarding.

4 PRESENTATION

"Your work is going to fill a large part of your life, and the only way to be truly satisfied is to do what you believe is great work. And the only way to do great work is to love what you do. If you haven't found it yet, keep looking, and don't settle. As with all matters of the heart, you'll know when you find it." – Steve Jobs

Now that productions are coming a town near you, you need to be prepared and ready for one of those movies or television shows to hire you. The goal is to gain enough experience in working with many types of people and their personalities before the productions hit your area. Envision yourself working in a trailer for a movie or spraying the fly-a-ways from a famous actor's head while onset. Keep your focus. Again, I began to prepare myself for the movie industry 20 years early unknowingly. This is why I can now help you line yourself up with your vision. While owning my salon I began teaching hair in the community colleges and being a platform artist with one of the leading hair companies. This helped to remove any fear of speaking to almost anyone and helped to teach me how to speak and answer questions without hesitation. All this that I was doing I realized under no circumstances I was doing exactly what I loved. I would eat, breathe and sleep the hair industry. This was my PASSION ! In order for you to do well, be successful and be happy you have to want it bad enough. It has to be your PASSION ! Take a moment close your eyes and ask yourself, "Do I eat, breathe, and sleep what I'm doing". If your answer is yes, well indeed it's your PASSION. Let's continue..

5 THE NEW HOLLYWOOD

"Change is inevitable, progress is optional." – Tony Robbins

There was a time when almost every production was shot in California but those days are gone. Just a few years ago I would not have considered putting this guide together to help other hairstylists or make-up artists learn how to become a film or television stylist. Why would I need to? Almost all the productions were right here in Hollywood.

I'm not sure if any of my other fellow union members were like me. I was in denial because I failed to recognize that productions were going away, and if they did come back it would never be the same and so far it hasn't been the same.

This realization took some time to get used to but then I realized that this change was going to take place whether we liked it or not! Because of the lack of knowledge on these "New Hollywood" crew sets there has been disasters after disasters and even fatalities. That's when I decided it's time to share because lives are being lost out there and if there's anything I can do to help my department prevent these tragedies I am willing to do it. So I'm deciding to share my experiences with you so that you can get on one of the sets in your area with a bit of knowledge that you didn't have before reading this book. #moretocomebook2

Some of you can achieve the dream that you've always wanted to right now in your own hometown. You no longer have to worry about moving to Hollywood. Your Hollywood is now right around the corner from you! So now you don't have to go far to prepare. My ultimate goal is to make sure that you're prepped and ready. I remember keying a film out of town and we had hundreds of background actors that we needed to get ready for production each day for 2 ½ months. Like all productions we hired locals and it was clear to me that they weren't ready. They were completely out of their element and that's simply because it wasn't something they had experience in. Doing hair and makeup for a photo shoot or fashion show is completely different from working on a movie set.

The locals were inexperienced when it came to timing, putting on wigs, adding facial hair, etc. It was a little frustrating to work with them because things needed to be very fast paced. Many hairstylist that come straight out of a salon to work on sets move at the salon pace and that's very slow. Not saying that the hairstylist isn't good at doing hair it's just on sets that's not the #1 importance. What is important is how much money you can save production and that means you have to be quick. After training one group of hairstylists and makeup artists we would have to train another group the next day because the first group couldn't all return. This was because they had clients at their salons or they had to work at makeup counters or maybe they wouldn't have a babysitter. The huge inconvenience cost the production a lot of money.

I want to help ensure that all hairstylists and makeup artists are ready for the movie and TV set. It is a very rewarding experience and I don't regret any of my time in the industry. In fact one of my passions is mentoring and helping others achieve great success within their fields using their creative artistic abilities. I'm writing this book because I've learned so much from working with the best in the business in a short period of time, and it was put on my heart to help you. I hope that through my knowledge and experience you will succeed in the now "New Hollywood"! Lights, Cameras...Alabama, Arizona, Arkansas, Kansas, Florida, Georgia, Idaho, Indiana, Iowa, Louisiana, Michigan, Mississippi,

Nebraska, Nevada, North Carolina, North Dakota, Oklahoma, South Carolina,

South Dakota, Tennessee, Texas, Utah, Virginia, Wyoming...Action!!!

6 ON MY OWN

"A ship is safe in harbor…but that's not what ships are for." –William Shedd

After having such a great teacher I decided I was ready to go out on my own. As I mentioned earlier, my motto in life is, "Always be a student". Never stop learning. Take as many classes as you can. Surround yourself with people that you can learn from. Be careful of the company that you keep. I remember one day hearing the re-known, Hip Hop Preacher, Eric Thomas say, "In order to be successful you have to be willing to give up sleep. Give up hanging at "Club Starbucks". Give up talking on your cell phone all day and night". He also said, "If you want to be successful, ask yourself how bad do you want it". It's not going to happen overnight but what he did say, at some point it's going to happen". What he says make lots of sense.

Let me give you an example of working hard. In an Olympic, Rowing setting, in the last 250 meters of the race, fighting for the bronze medal, it was time to put every bit of pain behind them. Instead of pushing harder in their boat as they watched the fourth place team start to overtake them, they began to sink back and let them win the bronze medal. If the rowers would have pushed harder and put pain and suffering before them, they would have been able to take home the bronze instead of watching someone else steal that from them. That is the way it works in life, too. If you don't want to suffer and put in the work you have to in order to be in a position where you're successful, you won't be, and you'll have to sit back and watch many people surpass you. Don't be that person. Take the initiative.

Ask questions, do your research, find the answers. Read, read, and read! This is where your inspiration and empowerment comes from. The harder you work, the more you know the more confidence you will have within yourself.

I went through four years of working in different salons, finding my niche, and trying to find where I could work in L.A. I finally found a salon right outside of Beverly Hills, a very thriving area of LA and it became home to me.

My clientele grew at a quick pace. I was referred a few celebrities, lots of high-end clients. I worked with directors, writers, actors, DJs, fitness trainers, and etc. Then one day, Garcelle Beauvais, my client at the time, referred Shaun Robinson from Access Hollywood to me. Garcelle Beauvais, actress, author and one of the pioneer African American fashion models of all time.

I began doing Shaun for all of her red carpets events, premieres, award shows, etc.. You name it and I was there with her. I was very faithful to my salon clients, and any hairstylists that has done hair for any length of time because of our loyalty will tell you that they don't want to leave their clients. Clients are very dear to us. They are our livelihood and they're our bread and butter. One day I had to make that one decision. Would I stay in the salon and work or should I work on sets behind the camera? Mind you, I still had three kids, so I was running around like a chicken with its head cut off. Going from the salon into the studios and back into the salon all within one day. I needed to make a decision about should I stay or go and my family was my first priority. So I made the decision to leave the salon. It was overall a more consistent and stable choice. Health insurance was at the top of my list for leaving. I had to look at it as a promotion.

Another question that I'm asked a lot is " how can I start doing hair on set?" Well here it is folks in a nutshell. I tell people all the time it's like a Catch 22. You have to have a working actor that can bring you into the studio to do their hair. My path was a straight line unlike most freelancers. I feel very blessed that my way of entering the union was by doing a union project. Most stylists have to do many non-union gigs to accumulate days to get into the union. I'm so very fortunate. Shaun and I have remained friends and I will always appreciate Shaun for our almost 7 years together that put me into the Hairstylists and Makeup Artists Union, Local 706. Thank you Ms. Robinson!

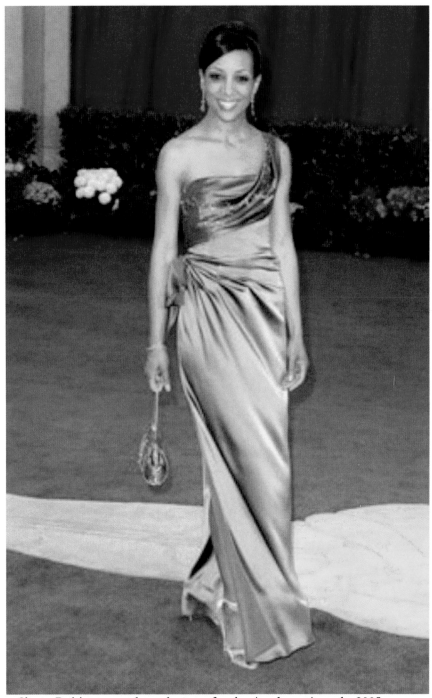

Shaun Robinson on the red carpet for the Academy Awards, 2005
Hair Styled by Rhonda O'Neal
Makeup by Val Hunt-Darden

7 KNOW YOUR WORTH

"If you don't know your own worth and value, don't expect someone else to calculate it for you." – Unknown

I again, have to refer back to my foundation in Texas and how I handled myself and my business is what drew this type of clientele to me. When you deal with high profilers always keep your focus. If you keep your focus on liking your clients, they will like you back and the way you act toward them will confirm that because they will keep coming to you. Know your worth because it is great to get high profilers for your clients but at the same time if they are coming to you, first you must be a wonderful person inside and out and then a great artist or whatever your profession is what's keeping them. Believe in yourself over anyone else. Don't try to keep up with them. Just be who you are. Don't put others before YOU. When you start doing that, the clients notice and they will begin treating you differently. Whenever, you have high regards for yourself people will always respect you. Okay, this doesn't mean once your clients come in and sit in your chair you start telling them all about your life and your woes. Some things you have to keep to yourself. Be discreet about what to talk about in regards to you. If you really focus on making your clients feel welcomed when you're with them, it will create ease.

If someone asked me to describe myself in five words I would say I'm compassionate, loving, loyal, humble and driven. Remember, know your worth. **Now, in five words describe yourself and write them down.**

1. _____

2. _____

3. _____

4. _____

5. _____

8 MY KEY TO SUCCESS

"I've always believed that if you put in the work, the results will come. I don't do things half-heartedly. Because I know if I do, than I can expect half-hearted results." -Michael Jordan

Would you believe me if I told you that 85% of my business has been through referrals? I've lived off of them for the last 30 years. This is why your reputation is everything. Your livelihood isn't just based off of how well you do hair. It will thrive according to how you treat and service people. You have to be able to build relationships. I say to almost everyone I meet, "The key to success is by building relationships one by one." Networking to me is not going to a function and collecting or handing out cards. That does nothing for me but clutter more junk on my desk, station or in my purse. I don't know any of those people that I just got a card from. But if I build a relationship with someone that person is more willing to help me if I've helped them with something or we've shared moments of pieces of our lives together. Be willing to do for others just because and greatness will come back to you. We work in an aesthetic service industry and clients are paying for an experience. You're not their friend. I'm not saying you can't become their friend but don't start by thinking you're going to make a friend out of them. Keep everything professional and the relationship will go a long way. Never forget that this is a business. However, when money is being exchanged, you have to know your place. You are their stylist and there is a level of professionalism that you have to exhibit at all times. With that being said, you have to gain the respect of people. From the beginning I realized that I didn't know how to do hair as well as some. When I first started, I worked for my mother. I got a lot of clientele because I was a great haircutter and stylist, but my mom was the business when it came to everything else. I would get the referrals of people for haircuts. So when I started seeing that, I thought, "Okay, people are coming to me, people must like what I'm doing."

So I started learning as much as I possibly could about hair. I flew to Chicago and took a Master class at the well renowned Pivot Point, and I sat under people that had owned and made their own products. They mentored me and taught me how and why they made their products and what made their products work better than others. I realized that the three people that I studied under were pharmacist before doing this. From that, I started gaining a lot of clients. I saw that people didn't just want to see how well I could do their hair, but they wanted to hear about how to keep their hair healthy when I wasn't around. People wanted to know about hair care, and they were thirsty for this knowledge. I'm the first to admit that I wasn't the best hairstylist and I wasn't the best creative hairstylist.

However, I taught my clients how to make their hair shiny and keep it healthy. That platform has stuck with me for my entire 30 something years.

That niche resulted in me getting clients from Houston to L.A. It finally dawned on me that I was good! I also noticed that my clients were extremely intelligent. I had to step my game up in terms of my knowledge. They were asking me questions as if I were a chemist. I needed to answer the questions in the same way that the people that I mentored under in Houston would have answered. I recalled a lot of the answers that they would give, and I started to regurgitate that information. During that time I learned everything that I could about hair and hair care. I became a platform artist for a one of the leading African American Hair Companies. I spoke and taught throughout the southern region of the US. I wanted the masses to learn hairstyling, haircutting but mainly hair care.

I stared doing Shaun Robinsons hair and she was just as knowledgeable. They were very well educated about their own hair. I said, "I have to make sure that I'm stepping up to the plate!" when you're working with those kinds of people, they learn so much about themselves. They are experts when it comes to their hair and skin. Celebrities do a lot of reading and research, so you have to be prepared and you can't be intimidated. When you're intimidated, you will sometimes get an attitude of, "I'm the hairstylist, don't try to tell me what to do!" Don't take on this attitude. When you're working with actors they learn so much about themselves during their auditioning days, when money was scarce and they couldn't afford to go to a salon every week they had to make do and they had to do it well.

So when they come to me, I love it! I love when I get celebrities because I don't have to work as hard because they already know what they want. All I have to do is help them keep up their image. Instead, a lot of hairstylists feel like they should tell celebrities what to do. When a celebrity gets into their chair they think it's the time to create a new image for them. This isn't the case. They've already established themselves, and they've worked hard to get to where they are. So we have to acquiesce to what they want us to do. That's really what our job is, servicing people. You can't have a "me" mentality when working with actors or any high-profiler. Take a backseat.

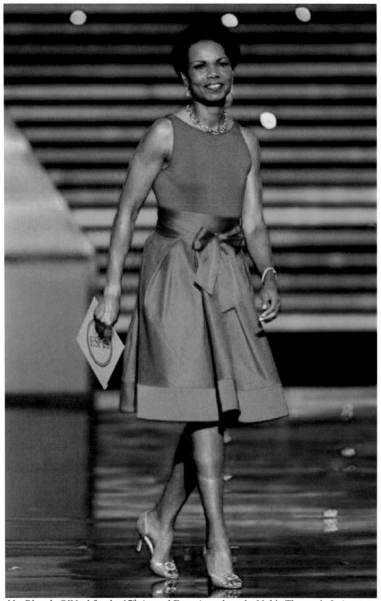
Hair Styled by Rhonda O'Neal for the 17th Annual Espy Awards at the Nokia Theater in L.A.

"One of my Aha moments and great example of a high-profiler and keeping my focus was when I got a call to do Condoleezza Rice's hair. Okay, the highest woman profiler in the United States. And if someone would ask me, when did you know you made it? My answer would be, I don't know if I will ever feel like I made it. There's always a new goal to strive for."

9 SOCIAL MEDIA

"We don't have a choice on whether we do social media, the question is how well we do it." –Erik Qualman

As an artist you have to use social media differently. I'm still trying to learn it more and more. I have a teenage daughter that knows more about it than I do. But when you decide to have Facebook and Instagram pages, you have to keep them professional. When you pass out your cards or teach a class, they will go directly to your social media profiles.

Do you really want them to know about the intricate details of your personal life? Do you think they want to know you were with #UncleBubba last night? LOL You can share, but some things you shouldn't post. If you absolutely have to share intimate moments online, then I suggest creating separate profiles.

Your social media should be filled with what your clients or potential clients and those that you're mentoring want to see.

That's just my quick two cents, you don't have to spend it if you don't want to. #imjustsaying

10 IT'S A WRAP!

"My mission in life is not merely to survive, but to thrive; and to do so with some passion, some compassion, some humor and some style". - Maya Angelou

Before we move on to the second portion of the book there are some thoughts that I would like to leave you with. Remember that the only limits that you have are the ones that you place on yourself. If you truly believe that you can't do something, then it becomes a self-fulfilling prophecy. Have faith and know that every client that sits in your chair is going to get you closer to your dream. Treat each one of them like royalty, and you can't go wrong.

The world is starving for new ideas, for YOUR new ideas. Learn the basics of the trade and unleash your creativity. Don't be afraid to try some of the ideas that you have. Fear is always going to be present but the key is to never give in. Ask the universe for what you want and know that it will answer. Stop playing it so safe! You can have a safe job or you can take a chance. You went into this industry because you like to think outside the box, go even further. You will get what others don't get by doing the things that others don't do. Salons are full of stylists that are still dreaming. It's your time to wake up and to make it happen. In case you're wondering, yes, this is a pep talk. So much of this journey is a mental one. I can tell you all of the tricks of the trade until I'm blue in the face but if you do not believe in yourself then it is pointless. You have a gift and it's time to share it with the world. Live your dream beyond the comb!

Celebrity

Hairstylist's

Guide to Success

GETTING STARTED

First and foremost as I mentioned you have to have a plan. Throughout this book, your main objective will be to create and finally set up your own plan for achieving your goals. I want to encourage you to think of Beyond the Combs as your workbook.

Create an environment of success by envisioning what your future can be like. Remove negative thoughts from your mind and replace them with words such as triumph, win, achieve, mission, defeat and happiness.

If you want to do something and you stick to it, it can be done. Stay focused and determined. If you need to get a part time job in order to survive at the beginning do it but don't let that discourage you. Sometimes in life we have to change our thinking in order for us to grow. This is one of those times. Don't restrict yourself to one type of thinking. Expand your mind. Sometimes we are set in our ways. New opportunities await you. This is where the increase comes from. Forward thinking. In other words, you're making room for growth and change. Clear away the weeds in your life and make room for amazing results. Think big. Think increase. Think wealth. Think more than enough. When you change the way you think you change your life. Think no more limitations. When you change your way of thinking so many doors will begin opening for you.

Back to my best friend and mentor (My mom, Mrs. B, may she rest in peace). She was a phenomenal teacher and I'm so glad I remember what she said from a long time ago because it is the bases of why I do, say, and teach the importance of hair and beauty. What she taught me has been invaluable. We have to realize if we get caught up in what we see it can cause us to lose focus on the bigger picture, which is WHY we really want to do hair, makeup or fashion in the world of entertainment.

Lesson #1: Ask yourself, why do you want to do red carpet events, photo shoots, television or film productions. Take a moment and write down why you want to come from behind the chair or whatever your job is.

How to build your portfolio

If you don't know any good professional photographers you can find them off of the internet. They are always looking for hairstylist to style their models for shoots. If you volunteer your expertise, in exchange they will give you tears for your portfolio.

You can search sites like Model Mayhem and Craigslist. Do an exchange with them. They're everywhere, and so this won't be a difficult opportunity to find. Just as much as you need them, they need you. Make sure to stay pleasant and professional throughout the shoot. Also follow up with the photographer to ensure that you get your shots.

Magazines are your friend. Look through magazines like Vogue, Elle, Harper's Bazaar, and etc. Talk to the photographer and ask him the direction of the shoot. Find out if it's a vintage, pinup, lifestyle, or commercial shoot. Do your research, look through a lot of magazines, tear out pictures, and bring them to the shoot. You can use those pictures as your inspiration.

How I Joined the Union

As mentioned before, in order to be able to come into the lot, you have to come onto the lot with an actress that is working on a show and can invite you onto their show. All actors aren't at the point where they can invite you. But those that are able to can bring you onto their show or movies with them. I was blessed that my actor was in a position to bring me on as her personal stylist.

So people wonder how to get on a set or in the union, and the only way to get in is to already have a celebrity client that's willing to bring you on set. It's such a catch 22, and that's why making the right connections are necessary. There is no other way. However, running around town and chasing down actors isn't the way to do it. They will be rude and treat you like you're paparazzi. They prefer to find you through a referral, a PR company, the studio, or the show that they're on.

I got into the union by the request of an actor on entertainment news. In entertainment news the requirement is that you have to go through the 60/60/60 rule. Which is 60 days for 3 years within a five year period. If I was working on a regular show or a movie, then the days are less.

Normally after the time of being on a network show or movie, if you're requested by an actor, you usually have accumulated the days that you need. There is also a fee that you must pay to the union. Now that they're so many right to work states you don't have to do the 60/60/60 rule. Call and ask your Film Commissioner at your state capital and they will refer you to who can give you the right information for your town.

Etiquette on Set

Your behavior while on set is the bases of you keeping a job in this industry. There's a lot going on once you get to the set. The actors, you the crew members are talking, laughing and appear to be really having a good time. Although that's truly the case you must always maintain your professionalism. Make sure you keep a watch of everything going on around you. There's always heavy equipment being moved around. Props and set dressing are moving furniture and some things are delicate. If the scene has weapons in it, this can be dangerous. These are some of the reasons you have to be well aware of your surroundings, so you won't get hurt.

I'm always asked if an intern can shadow me and unfortunately I have to tell them no. If I was working in a salon this wouldn't be a problem. Since I work on sets, this just isn't possible for me.

The unions are extremely private. The sets, lots, and trailers are the actor's home away from home. They are there over 16 hours a day and we're they're family. They have to feel comfortable, so there isn't any way that an intern could come on to the set. On most sets now visitors are limited to 15 minutes, and some sets don't allow anyone at all.

Sets have been shut down because people haven't abided by these rules. It's a job and it has to be treated as such.

Discussion Questions

Have you ever imagined yourself accomplishing your dreams? Do you keep the vision of success in front of you? How do you describe yourself?

Write down your dreams that you wish this book would help you accomplish.

Now describe what your life might look like when those dreams begin coming true.

Ask yourself, why do you want to do red carpet events, photo shoots, and television or film productions. Take a moment and write down why you want to come from behind the chair or whatever your current job is.

Stay Humble

"Humble enough to know I'm not better than anybody & wise enough to know that I'm different from the rest." - Unknown

It's so simple to get caught up in the lavish lifestyle. You have the amazing job of working with celebrities and you're responsible for their image. That must mean that you're a celebrity too right? NO, it doesn't. I don't want to knock anyone off of their high horse, but I urge you to remain humble if you want to continue in this industry and get more work. The sky's the limit to you!

They're more likely to re-hire the humble stylist that's easy to work with than the stylist that has the, "I'm the diva attitude." At the end of the day, that's what you really want right? To make money and live wonderfully.

"The highest calling of leadership is to unlock the potential of others". - Carly Fiorina.

SAMPLE

FORMS

&

WORK

SHEETS

Front of Call Sheet

Crew Call

Use the correct piece of equipment for the job

7A

| Shooting Call | 730A |

Executive Producer	Rhonda O'Neal	Thursday September 13, 2014
Co-Executive Producer	Terry O'Neal , II	Shoot Day: 4 of 5
Supervising Producer	Te'Rhon O'Neal	Weather High 83° Low 63°
Producer	Tyra O'Neal	Sunny 0% Chance of Rain
Writer	Rhonda O'Neal	Sunrise: 607A Sunset:751P

"It's Your Time"

Production#: 01002

Closed Set, No Visitors Without Prior Approval! No Personal Photography Allowed Onset!

Nearest Hospital: Celebrity Hospital 4428 Combs Ave. Hollywood, CA 90022

Production Office: (213) 555-5555

SET DESCRIPTION	SCENE	CAST	D/N	PGS	LOCATION
Interior Rhonda's House	12	1,2	D2	1	Quail Valley
Exterior Hair Masters Beauty Salon	2	1,2,4	D1	1	FM2234

#	CAST	CHARACTER	STATUS	REH	MU/HAIR	READY	NOTES
1	Rhonda O'Neal	Sasha	W		530A	7A	
2	Tyra O'Neal	TyTy	W		530A	7A	Fitting First
3	Terry O'Neal, II	Tbone	H	O	L	D	
4	Te'Rhon O'Neal	Tbaby	SWF		630A	7A	Haircut First

CONTINUITY SHEET

ACTOR_____ CHARACTER_____

PHOTO	PHOTO	PHOTO	PHOTO
1	2	3	4

Basic Description_____

Coloring_____

Wigs_____

Facial Hair_____

Hair Pieces_____

Hair Spray_____

Gel_____

Pomade_____

Curlers_____

Irons_____

Hairstyle_____

Products_____

Hair Length_____

Hair Style_____

Other_____

HAIR NOTES

Title:_____ Episode #_____ Sc. Day_____

Actor Character

Notes:

_____
_____
_____
_____
_____
_____
_____
_____
_____
_____
_____.

PHOTOS:

Glossary

Glossary

1ST ASSISTANT DIRECTOR (1ST AD): Assists the Director in setting the shot and scheduling

1ST ASSISTANT CAMERAMAN: Responsible for camera and camera crew working well. Assists operator pulling focus on camera for a shot.

2ND ASSISTANT DIRECTOR (2ND AD): Assists 1st AD in setting shot, setting extras, makes call sheets, handles paperwork for production report.

2ND ASSISTANT CAMERAMAN: Responsible for camera equipment, loading of film and slate.

2ND ASSISTANT DIRECTOR: Assists in crowd and traffic control, helps with background extras.

CREW CALL: The time the crew comes into work. Hair, make-up, wardrobe are called in up to 2 hours (sometimes more for FX make-up) then the rest if the crew.

AD: Abbreviation for Assistant Director
Also see 1st Assistant and 2nd Assistant Director.

ACADEMY AWARDS: Honors the work for artistic and technical achievements in many areas of Motion Pictures. This award is given to the members of the academy of Motion Pictures Arts and Sciences.

ACADEMY OF MOTION PICTURES ARTS AND SCIENCES (AMPAS): This is an honorary organization of filmmakers. Membership with AMPAS is by invitation only from the members in the academy. You must have feature film credits and years in the business to back-up your art.

ACCOUNTING CLERK: Postings.

ACCOUNTING: The staff that processes time cards, payroll, accounts receivables and payables.

ACTION: Movement of the camera, co-coordinated with actor movement.

ADR: Abbreviation for Automatic Dialogue Replacement.

AFI: Abbreviation for the American Film Institute.

AFM: Abbreviation for American Federation of Musicians.

AFTRA: Abbreviation for American Federation of Television and Radio Artists.

AGENCY: An office with staff comprised of agents.

AGENT: Person or company licensed by the state to represent clients and negotiate contracts on their behalf. The standard agents fee is ten percent of the clients salary.

AMPAS: Abbreviation for Academy of Motion Picture Arts and Sciences.

APPLE BOX: Standard size wooden crate used to raise the height of people, lights, or props during shooting. Apple boxes come in half and quarter sizes.

ART DEPARTMENT: Crew members who, under the direction of the Production Designer, are responsible for creating the look of a film as far as Sets on stage or a location.

ART DIRECTOR: Works with the Director overseeing the "look" of the film. Supervises building and dressing of the sets. Art directors must be knowledgeable in architecture and design. A very visual job.
ASSISTANT EXTRAS COORDINATOR: Helps wrangles extras.

ASSISTANT PRODUCTION CONTROLLER: Disbursement of paychecks.

ASSIST SET DECORATOR: Works with the set decorator preparing the sets.

ASSIST WARDROBE DESIGNER: Works w/the designer in the selection of the wardrobe for the cast.

ATMOSPHERE: Groups of people who fill in the spaces of the scene. Also known as Background Atmosphere/Artist.

AUDITION: The actor's reading or test for playing a character in a play or movie.

AVAILABLE LIGHT: Shooting with the natural light available. No added artificial light.

BACK LOT: This is an area at studios where sets are free standing. These can be a western town, major city streets such as New York and Chicago, or futuristic looking building.

BASE CAMP: The main location where all the trailers of company park.

BEST BOY GRIP: Assists key grip in running the department, ordering supplies, etc.

BEST BOY: 1st assist to the gaffer. Supervises laying the cables and he electrical crew.

BG: Abbreviation for Background.

BLOCKING: Laying out the action or movement in a scene with the actor and camera department. Also, placement of lighting.

BLUE-SCREEN/GREEN-SCREEN: A delicate and elaborate special effects process whereby the subject is filmed in front of a special, monochromatic blue or green background with normal film. Blue or green sensitive mattes are made to replace the blue or green background with other footage. When combined, the subject and background look as if they were shot simultaneously. Flying scenes and water scenes are usually shot like this.

BOOK: A diary of your past work.

BOOKING: Getting a job.

BOOM OPERATOR: The boom man holds the microphone on the end of a pole so that it is in the optimum position to record the dialogue of a scene. A good boom operator understands how the set runs, lighting, camera angles and the frame of a shot.

BOX RENTAL: a daily or weekly sum paid to a crew member for the use of his or her personal equipment during production.

BUDGET: Amount of money you get to spend on a show.

BUDGET LIST: A list of all expenses possible. The budget list cannot be made until the script is read, and it can be change during filming, due to script changes.

BURN OUT: When you work too hard and need a rest from the business.

CABLE MAN: Assists the boom operator and holds a second microphone when necessary.

CAKE WALK: Very easy job.

CALL SHEET: This is the work sheet that is prepared by the 2nd AD, approved by the 1st AD, then approved and signed by the production manager. On this sheet are the times for each crew member and actor and the scenes that will be shot that day. It also has a map to the set location for the day.

CALL TIME: This is the time you are to report to work.

CALLBACK: When an actor returns to audition for a role for a second or more times.

CAMEO: A small role played by a well-known actor to boost the ratings of the show.

CAMERA ANGLE: The point of view (POV) of the camera when it is set up to shoot a scene.

CAMERA OPERATOR: Manually operates camera during shooting.

CAMERA: Holds the film.

CARRY DAY/ON HOLD: A day the actors/crew are paid but not required to work.

CAST LIST: A list of actor's agent and manger's home number and address.

CASTING AGENT: Coordinates casting and talent, and negotiations of actors' contracts.

CASTING DIRECTOR: This person is responsible for casting the actors. It's always good to stay in contact with the casting director to get a picture of the actors you'll be working with also to be able to pull a wig if need be.

CASTING: Finding, selecting and signing actors.

CHARACTER NUMBER: This is a number assigned to an actor/character for the call sheet and production board. the lower the number, the bigger the actor.

CHECK THE GATE: It is the responsibility of the 1st assist cameraman to look down the camera lens and check if any hair or fuzz is present in the gate of the camera. This is usually done after a scene is complete.

CLIENT: The person for whom you are working.

CLOSE-UP (CU): A view of the actors up close in a scene.

CLOSED-SET: This is when only the crew members are allowed on set. If an intimate scene is being shot, only the crew member necessary to shoot the scene will be allowed on set.

COMMISSARY: The cafeteria on a studio lot.

COMPOSITE: A card with pictures of your work.

CONCEPT MEETING: Getting creative ideas together for the look of the show. Also, discussing certain scenes and how they will get shot.

CONSTRUCTION CREW: Crew member who, under the supervision of the construction foreman, perform the tasks necessary to complete the sets in and out of the studio. The crew is made up of the prop makers, painters and laborers

CONTINUITY: It is the hairstylist's job to keep the consistency of the look of the hair take after take. It is the script supervisor's job to keep the continuity of the action in the scene take after take.

COVER SET: An alternate film location and timetable which can be used in the event that shooting cannot proceed as planned. Often, exterior shooting is thwarted by weather, so it is imperative to have a backup schedule of interior shooting which can be substituted. It's also we say to each other when we need to go to the restroom or leave to do another actor. We say, "will you cover set for me while I'm gone".

COVERAGE SHOOTING: scenes from all different angles

CRAFT SERVICE: The department that serves foods to the crew throughout the day.

CREDITS: The list of cast and crew member listed at the end of a movie.

CREW LIST: A list of the crew with address and phone numbers. Keep this list so you can call people from it to stay abreast of upcoming productions.

CUT: A tern used by the director when he/she wants to stop the acting/action in a scene.

DP: Abbreviation for Director of Photography.

DAY PLAYER: An actor who only has a couple of lines in the movie

DEAL MEMO: A legal contract you have with production outlining your pay and the type of contract you're working under.

DEFERRED PAYMENT: Some low budget movies will have deal memo stating that your payment for working on the movie will be a percentage of how much the movie makes at the box office.

DEPARTMENT HEAD: The boss.

DGA: Abbreviated for Directors Guild of America.

DIALOGUE COACH: A member of the crew that helps the actors with their lines or accents.

DIRECTOR OF PHOTOGRAPHY: The person responsible for visually setting the shot and lighting.

DOLLY GRIP OPERATES: the camera dolly during the shot.

DOUBLE STICK TAPE: Tape that is sticky on both sides. Used for toupees and wardrobe.

DOUBLE: A person who looks like the actor. Also called, body double, stunt double and photo double

DRESS REHEARSAL: to rehearse a scene in costume

DRESSERS: Responsible for making sure the actors costumes are in their dressing rooms and, assisting the actors with dressing

EDITOR: Works closely with the director editing the film, and runs the editing room.

ELECTRICAL DEPARTMENT: The department which handles set lighting.

ELECTRICIANS: Crew that physically works with cable and lights setting the lights for the shot.

EMMY: An award for your great work in television from the ACADEMY of TELEVISION ARTS and SCIENCE. Voted on by Academy members.

ESTABLISHING SHOT: Also known as EXTREME LONG or MASTER SHOT. The camera sees everything in the scene. The lens on the camera is usually a wide angle lens. What this means to a hairdresser is that on screen, the actors are usually very small and you don't see much detail on the hair style, so make sure the shape of the style is in good form and relax. When they go in for coverage on the scene, then you will be needed to keep the hair in place.

EXPENDABLES: Hair spray, gel products, hair pins, and other things that get used up and need replacing.

EXPENSES: Purchases needed for the show.

EXT: Abbreviation for Exterior. A scene shot outside.

EXTRAS COORDINATOR: Finds and handles extras.

EYE LINE: This is a very important term to know. This term means being in the actor's eye line, where they can see you, when they are acting their scene. Some actors do not want you to be in their eye line.

FALL: Half of a wig that sits on the crown of the head.

FEATURE ACTORS: Whichever group of actors the camera sees the most in the scene.

FEATURE: Seen in the movie theater. A full length film is a minimum of 85 minutes long.

FILM MAKER: Everyone that works on a movie, no matter what you do, is a film maker. All jobs help with the making of a film.

FISH EYE: To a person in the camera department, this would be considered a camera lens. (An extremely wide angle lens causes a distorted image). To a department head in hair or make-up, this is the look you get from the UPM when they want you to release some of your extra help for the day.

FITTING: Measuring the actor for a wig or hair piece.

FLASHBACK: A scene that takes you back in time.

FLASH FORWARD: A clip in the scene where the audience gets to look into the future of what might happen to the actor.

FLASHING: Before taking a continuity picture on set, you'll yell, "FLASHING" so the lighting department can hear you and they don't think a light is burning out.

FLAT RATE: A set salary rate with no overtime.

FOG MACHINE: A special effect of smoke to make the lighting look soft and moody. In my opinion, the stuff stinks and you can't breathe for a couple days afterward. It's like being in a Smokey night club without alcohol to numb the senses.

FRAME: What the camera sees in the shot.

FREELANCER: An independent contractor.

GAFFER: Head of the electrical department. Works with the Director of Photography setting the lights or shadows.

GETTING YOUR TURN AROUND: For stage work, the union has made a rule that a crew member must get nine hours of rest before coming back to work the next day. The rule is ten hours when you work on location. If you do not get the proper TURN AROUND TIME, you are on TIME & A HALF until you hit hour nine or ten hours, whichever applies. *See TIME & A HALF.*

GOLDEN TIME/ DOUBLE TIME: This makes everyone happy but production. After you have worked 12 hours in a day, your salary doubles; otherwise known as DOUBLE TIME or GOLDEN TIME.

GAFFER'S TAPE: This is simply duct tape with a lot of purpose.

GREENSMAN: The person responsible for all the plants on set. If you're lucky, you may get a plant or two to take home.

GRIP: The electricians put lights up and the grips move walls or anything that is not a prop. They also lay dolly track for the camera and move the dolly with the camera on it.

HAIR STYLIST: Usually a licensed cosmetologist styling the actor's hair or wig to create the look of the character. Department head hair makes the decisions, and the assistant helps perform the duties in the department.

HIATUS: Television shows shut down for one week to three months. This gives everyone on the crew time to relax before starting up again.

HOLLYWOOD CLAUSE: In a written agreement, the Hollywood Clause states that your agent does not get a cut of your pay for jobs you get on your own.

HONEYWAGON: This is a truck that has rest rooms and rooms for the cast to get dressed. On location, production will make one of the rooms and office.

HOT SET: This is a set where the scene has not been completed and all the props are in place and can not be moved. This way they can pickup filming where they left off.

I.A.T.S.E: Abbreviation for International Alliance of Theatrical and Stage Employees. The parent organization of at least 1,000 local unions in North America.

ID: The camera department uses a slate to record the scene number, name of the show, director, DP, and number of scene takes. This helps the editors keep track of the scenes when editing.

INCIDENTALS and TRANSPORTATION: Additional monies you receive when you go on location.

IN THE CAN: Film that has been processed from a move camera is in a tin can shaped like the reel. When all the shooting happens to prevent a scheduled day of shooting. (e.g., bad weather, injury to an actor, earthquake, fire, etc.)

INT: Abbreviation for Interior. A scene shot inside.

KEY GRIP: Head of the grip department.

KEY: The First Assistant to the department head of hair or make-up.

KIT FEE: Reimbursement for expendables and renting of your equipment.

LACE FRONT: Lace around the edges of a wig to make it look natural to the camera's eye.

M.O.W.: Movie of the Week.

MAGIC HOUR: The time between sundown and darkness.

MAKE-UP ARTIST: A qualified artist hired to apply make-up to create the look of a character an actor is playing. In this department there is a department head that runs the department and makes the decisions, and an assistant.

MATTES: Are used in Special Effects for combining separate images onto one piece of film, changing backgrounds or the tons of an image.

MERKIN: A patch of hair that resembles hair on the groin area.

MILEAGE: If your job location is ten miles away from the production office's door, and you drive your vehicle to the location. You will get paid MILEAGE.

MOS: Abbreviation for MIC OUT SOUND. Camera roles film and sound will not record.

NABET: Abbreviation for National Alliance of Broadcast Engineers and Technicians. Union for commercials and some television.

NEWBIES: Someone new to the film business.

NO QUOTE DEAL: When negotiating a deal memo, you can request that the amount of your deal will not get quoted to anyone in the industry. (This is useful on low budget films, so no one knows what you were paid on the film).

NOTICE OF CANCELLATION: As a courtesy, the company should give you a 24 hour notice of cancellation or you can charge them (something to have in your contract).

OC: Abbreviation for OFF CAMERA.

ON A BELL: On a sound stage at the studios, outside the entrance door to the stage, there's a red light and a bell that rings to let people know not to enter the stage while rolling.

ON-CALL: This is when you are put on hold and will be called later when you are needed to return to work.

OVER THE SHOULDER: Camera is looking over the actor's shoulder on to another person.

OVERTIME: Money paid to your for working over 8 hours.

P.A.: Abbreviation for Production Assistant. The hardest working person on a crew and the lowest paid.

PER DIEM: This is extra food money you receive when you go on location.

PERIOD PIECE: Count twenty years back from today's date and that's a period piece.

PICKUP: Pickup up on a take so that the director can see if he can get better acting from the actor.

PILOT: This is a sample of a television program which production companies film and attempts to sell to a network as a show that is scheduled as a weekly program. Otherwise known as episode television or situation comedy.

POST-PRODUCTION: Wrapping up production, editing film, closing the office.

PRE-CALL: A time before crew call when some of the crew can prepare their job before the day's work begins.

PREP: Getting organized for a show.

PRE-PRODUCTION: The organization of a production before the first day of shooting principal photography.

PRINCIPAL PHOTOGRAPHY: The first day of shooting the movie.

PRINCIPAL PLAYERS: The actors featured in a scene.

PRINT: This is the take of the scene the director likes. The script supervisor makes a note of it in his or her script notes and the editor gets these notes and knows which take to PRINT of a scene.

PROP ASSISTANT: Usually works the set making sure that the correct props are on set for each scene.

PROP DEPARTMENT: Anything held by a actor or moveable on a table is an prop.

PROP MASTER: Responsible for the selection, rental or purchase of all props used in the film and the management of the department.

PRODUCTION ASSISTANT: Utility gofer. A perfect entry spot if you don't know what you want to do in the film business. *See P.A.*

PRODUCTION CONTROLLER: Budget management.

PRODUCTION COORDINATOR: Works with UPM on logistics of production.

PRODUCTION MEETING: The Director meets with the crew to discuss how he or she wants to the shoot the movie.

PRODUCTION REPORT: The Assistant Director's document the days work on a report called a PRODUCTION REPORT.

PRODUCTION SECRETARY: Handles office correspondence.

PRODUCTION: A group of film makers working together to make a movie.

PUBLICISTS: A person that works for you to help put you in the public eye.

PURCHASE ORDER NUMBER: A PO number is the number of the invoice you get from production when ordering supplies for the show.

QUIET ON THE SET/ QUIET PLEASE: The most expressed phrase an AD shouts to quiet the crew down before rolling the camera.

RE-DRESS: Settling the props back to the original procession from the top of the scene.

RE-SHOOT: Re-shooting a scene or scenes because something in the previous shoot went wrong or there was a change to the script.

REEL: An example of your work to use in interviews.

REVISIONS: Rewrites of a script.

ROLLING: The ADs announce this out loud to the crew when the camera is about to roll film.

ROUGH CUT: A rough edited version of a film.

RUSHES/ DAILIES: These are the clips of work shot the day before for the viewing pleasure of the Director, D.P Hair, Make-Up, Actor, Gaffer, Producer, Wardrobe, etc.

SAG: Abbreviation for Screen Actor's Guild.

SAND BAG: A bag filled with sand to act as a weight to anchor or hold an object steady.
SCENE: The script is broken-down into scenes.

SCRIPT BREAKDOWN: Separating each and every element of the script. If there are action and stunts required, you may need a wig. If there's a time lapse in a scene, or a different day in a scene, this could mean a hair change. Breakdowns keep all this organized for these shooting days.

SEAMSTRESS: Responsible for the sewing and repair of costumes.

SERIES: Referred to as Episodic Television. A mini-movie shot in eight days. Thirteen to twenty-one episodes are shot in a series.

SET DECORATOR: Responsibility for dressing the set with furniture relevant to the various scenes.

SET DESIGNER: The person responsible for planning the construction of the sets, from the description and drawings of the ART DIRECTOR/ PRODUCTION DESIGNER.

SET DRESSERS: These people work ahead of the crew dressing the sets and getting the look right for upcoming scenes.

SET: The place where all the action happens.

SHOOT DAY: A day the camera roles and everyone works.

SHOOTING SCHEDULE: A breakdown of the scenes in the script, when they're going to be shot and the location with the names of the characters working.

SHOT: A continuous take of a scene; a scene the camera shoots.

SINGLE: The camera only sees one actor in the shot, or something that works best when working in this business (being single).

SOUND DEPARTMENT: Usually a three-person crew consisting of the Sound Mixer, Boom Operator and the Cable Puller. Then there is the Post Production Mixer who mixes all the tracks when the picture is cut together.

SOUND MIXER: Runs the actual recording machine and as head of the department, decides on the overall approach on how to mic the scene.

SOUND STAGE: A stage on a studio lot.

SOUND EDITOR: Edits and creates the sound effects for the movie. This department also has an assistant position.

SPECIAL EFFECTS: An exciting but very dangerous department. They handle firearms, explosives, bullets hits, rain, smoke, and any kind of effect to make the scene more believable. This department has a coordinator and an assistant.

SPEED: The sound department is recording sound.

SPIRIT GUM: Glue used on the skin to adhere lace, prosthetics, etc.

STAND-IN: A person that stands in for the actor while the camera and lighting departments do their jobs.

STATE RIGHT-TO-WORK: Laws make these make these sorts of contracts illegal, **meaning** workers in unionized businesses can benefit from the terms of a union contract without paying union dues.

STEADICAM: A vest that straps the camera to the cameraman.

STERADICAM OPERATOR: Operates special hand held camera mounts.

STILL PHOTOGRAPHER: Usually a one man department that takes action shots of scenes to be used to advertise the show.

STINGER/ CABLE: A long extension cord for electricity to give power to the lights.

STRAIGHT TIME: Your salary for an eight hour day is STRAIGHT TIME.

STRIKE A SET: Take everything down and go home.

SW: Abbreviation for START WORK. Meaning the first day of the actor's work.

SWF: Abbreviation for START WORK FINISH. Meaning the actor is only working for one day.

T-PIN: A needle like pin formed like a "T" to help block a wig.

TAKE: A continuous shot of a scene made by the camera. A director may want many takes before he or she sees what they want for the scene. Rolling the camera to a shoot a scene is a TAKE.

TALENT: Actor's and animals are called TALENT.

TEARSHEET: Published and credited work in a magazine.

TESTING: A practice run with the actor doing hair and make-up to see what it looks like on film.

THE MARTINI: Referred to as the last shot of the day. Back in the day, when a film crew wrapped around happy hour, everyone went out for a drink. So, the last shot of the day was nick named, "THE MARTINI".

TIME & A HALF: Your salary wage plus half more. For example, $10.00/hour plus half is $5.00 equaling $15.00/hour. This wage is paid between eight hours and ten hours of work. After ten hours you're in double time. YIPPEE...

TOASTMASTER: A group of people from different professions getting together to master mind and support each other in being the "best you can be".

TOP BILLING: The opening credits at the beginning of a film will have one name listed (TOP BILLING) before another name. A well-known actor or crew person, producer(s) and writers will have this negotiated into their contract.

TOUPEE: A crown wig for a man.

TRAILER: Clips of a film for advertising purposes is a TRAILER.

TRAINEE, DGA: An Assistant Director doing on the job training through a program sponsored by the DGA. (DIRECTORS GUILD ASSOCIATION). It is imperative to let the AD TRAINEE know how important it is to work in harmony with Hair and Make-Up. AD TRAINEES will bring the actors to you in the morning to get ready, and to you for after lunch touch-ups.

TRANSPORTATION DEPARTMENT: Responsible for all vehicles working on or in the picture. In this department there is the Coordinator who runs the department, rents vehicles and hires the drivers. The Transportation Captain assists the Coordinator , organizing where the trucks will be parked on location, and stage locations, and the van drivers that transport the crew from crew parking to base camp, and to the set's location.

TRAVEL DAY: A paid day for traveling to a distant location.

TURNING AROUND: The camera is moved to the other side of the room, when the scene is completely shot in that angle. "TURN AROUND" meaning shoot the scene from the other direction.

UNIT PRODUCTION MANAGER: Head of production, oversees all aspects of the filming.

VENTILATED: Strands of human hair hand tied on a net cap. This process is used in wig making.

VIDEO VILLAGE: This is the Director, Script Supervisor, and DP's office. It is an area on set where monitors are present for the viewing pleasure of the scene being shot with the camera.

WARDROBE DEPARTMENT: This department is responsible for all the costumes worn in the movie. This department works very close with Hair and Make-Up.

WARDROBE DESIGNER: Works closely with the director in deciding on the look of the show and then supervises his or her crew in the purchase, rental or creation of the costumes.

WEFT: Abbreviation for WORK FINISHED. Meaning the last day the actors work.

WIG BLOCK: A head form to put a wig on.

WIG CAP: A stocking hat put on the head to hold hair under a wig.

WIG STAND: A metal clamp to hold a wig block.

WIGLET: A small wig that covers a bald patch on the head.

WRAP: The director calls this out when the day of shooting is finished. "IT'S A WRAP!"

ABOUT THE AUTHOR

Entering into the hair industry with her mother, Barbara Curtis Stroman (Mrs. B), Rhonda Stroman O'Neal, took over the scene becoming one of Houston's sought after hairstylists. Rhonda attended Franklin Beauty School, and later Chicago's Pivot Point. She's taught in the Houston Community Colleges, worked as a Platform artist for major hair companies and has been a mentor to several now great artists. She also helped to motivate her 2 sisters to go to beauty school and become wonderful hairstylists in their own right. At the mere age of 21, Rhonda opened her own salon and employed 10 hairstylists for nearly 10 years. The cool part is that her employees never left her side until she sold it and moved to Los Angeles. While in Texas, Rhonda did hair for high-profilers and athletes and their wives, the Miss Black Texas and Miss Texas pageants, local news and cable shows.

She grew up in the 70's when the oil business was booming in Texas. Many families were being relocated there. Moving into the plush gated communities those people became her clients. Surprisingly enough the oil began to dry up and those families were being laid off and couldn't come to the salon like consistently. At that moment Rhonda realized she needed to begin a new work within herself. She knew the loss of those clients and the drop in her business was only temporary. Rhonda tends to look at life and obstacles a bit differently. The struggle may last a day or even a year but eventually it would be over. It may be painful but pain is temporary and she knows if she quits however, it will last a lifetime.

Rhonda began teaching in the Houston Community Colleges and worked as a Platform artist for major hair companies. Rhonda's mission now is to help teach others what she was so fortunate to receive from her mom. To Rhonda, foundation is key. If you don't have a good foundation than it's hard to set your stage. The knowledge she received from Mrs. B the student's coming out of beauty school today will never receive. That's what one would call "Old School Knowledge", defined as knowledge you can't find in a textbook. Rhonda will tell you her mom taught her "HAIR" not hairstyling but hair in its essence. Her mom worked back in the 1960's when colored folks weren't allowed to step foot in a white salon but Mrs. B worked in one of the exclusive neighborhoods of Houston known as "River Oaks" comparable to Beverly Hills as their "shampoo girl". Mrs. B was their "Colorist" and boy was she a colorist. She taught Rhonda everything from hair coloring to hair straightening. Mrs. B taught Rhonda the meaning of hair from how to grow it to how to maintain it.

The knowledge she received from her mom has been invaluable. Till this day she credits her mom, for everything. She is so grateful for listening and absorbing what her mom had to offer her. Sometimes she ask herself now that Mrs. B is gone did she miss something or forget something she may have said during her days hanging out in her mom's salon where she learned, listened and absorbed? Rhonda always credits her success to all of her mentors that taught her that information changes situations. She began taking as many classes as she could to learn everything about hair. Rhonda learned many years ago that the best way to becoming successful is by, setting the atmosphere. She became obsessed with improvement. She spent more time sitting under people, going to conferences and asking questions. When Rhonda mentors others she reminds them to never stop being a student. It doesn't matter if you're 5 or 55 be a student. Always be willing to learn.

Being successful to Rhonda is being able to give up sleep. Give up hanging at "Club Starbucks". Give up talking on your cell phone all day and night. Speaking of cell phones we're a consumer based society. We have to always get the next upgrade of technology. But we're not upgrading ourselves. We're the same

operating system from 1990 as we were in 2010, still talking and thinking the same. But I guarantee all of your computers, TV's, telephones and cars have been upgraded. We're consumers more than producers. We spend more money than we are making. We have to begin focusing our mind on buying a book rather than the latest purse or buying an online class instead of the latest cell phone.
Focus is key…from the words of Eric Thomas, "If you want to be successful, ask yourself how bad do you want it".
It's not going to happen overnight but at some point it's going to happen.

Once Rhonda moved to LA and began making her mark in Hollywood, she began receiving referrals from high-profilers once more and this time actors instead of athletes. One being Shaun Robinson, a reporter on Access Hollywood referred by actress/model, Garcelle Beavauis. From that appointment as a hairstylist Rhonda's life changed. Shaun needed her at the studio, on the red carpet, at junkets, everywhere Shaun went, she needed her hair to look good all the time. Rhonda was her girl. This was the dream of a lifetime job for any hairstylist. She met almost every celebrity that works in the entertainment industry. At the time she had no idea all these days were going toward getting into the Hairstylists and Makeup Artists Union. Rhonda was a mom not thinking of anything but helping to feed her family. She didn't seek after being in the union it sought after her.

As a hairstylist with already over 20 years in the business Rhonda didn't know there was more for her to learn about hair and this business. She received her days in the union what's called 60/60/60 and that allowed her the opportunity to work on union run television shows and films. After six years of what she calls "Her Access Hollywood Family" it was time for her to go into the "Real Hollywood" where union productions were being made. One Sunday she attended a union meeting and was in conversation with a young lady that started asking her what she was doing at the time and Rhonda told her, working on Access

Hollywood. The very next day she got a call to offer her the Key position of a TV show and after careful consideration being a wife and mother of 3 Rhonda took the job because it was more money and better benefits for her family.

Rhonda is known as the "Healthy Hair Guru". Her approach for each client is to thoroughly assess their hair which helps to build the framework for a lasting relationship. Whether it's for a long-term client or for a season on a TV show or for a few weeks on a movie. The information one receives to revive or enhance their hair works and is unique to what any stylist does. One of the greatest compliments Rhonda received was from NCIS:LA actress Daniela Ruah. She mentioned as a child actress and in all of her years of working day after day on set her hair has never been this healthy." Working every day and given Rhonda's daily hair regimen my hair looks and feels better than it ever has".

This is what distinguishes Rhonda from her peers. This is what certifies Rhonda as a master stylist and hair care specialist. When you sit in Rhonda's chair whether in the salon or in the trailer Rhonda will give you her own "Hair Regimen" that you will be instructed to do and after however many weeks Rhonda instructs you to do you will than see amazing results. Rhonda has called it her very own "Cocktail" for many years. From her careful instructions to revive her high profile client's hair her list became longer and longer. From busy moms to A-list actors, athletes, musicians to political figures, because of her knowledge of hair and her, what one would say about a doctor her "bedside manners", for that reason alone it has acquired her so many loyal clients over the years. Rhonda has done hair for every Awards show from the Oscars, to the Golden Globe to the People's Choice to the Grammys to the Screen Actors Guild to the BET Awards. She has done hair for several films and television shows such as "Brooklyn Nine Nine", "Hit the Floor", "Eagleheart", "Argo", "Gangster Squad", "Pirates of the Caribbean", "Indiana Jones", " John Hancock", "Star Trek", " NCIS:LA", "90210", "One on One", "Dancing With The Stars", and "Modern Family". Her list of clients includes Laila Ali, Cybill Shepherd, Mila Kunis, Jason Bateman,

Todd Smith (LL Cool J), Salli Richardson, Daniela Ruah, Solange Knowles, Free, Roshumba Williams, Eric Andre, Chelsea Peretti, Andre Braugher, and Condoleezza Rice. Rhonda's work has been seen in magazines such as Vogue, Bazaar, Black Hairstyles, People, Flaunt, and TV Guide. Rhonda has done the BET Awards since its inception and in 2013 was given the honor of becoming Beauty Director for the BET Experience "My Black is Beautiful" Covergirl/Pantene Campaign sponsored by Proctor and Gamble. And has been offered the opportunity again in 2014.

Give Rhonda a client from any walk of life and she guarantees they'll have an unmatched and incomparable hair experience of a lifetime. That client will leave Rhonda with knowledge unheard of sure to benefit their hair for years to come. Rhonda is at the peak of her life and very happy where she is and even more happy for where she's headed!

"It's when I turn my client to the mirror and I see their eyes…a sense of peace come over them because they feel like they are now with someone they can trust. A confidence even the eyes can't hide."

Rhonda O'Neal

#ILoveWhatIDoAndIDoWhatILove

www.BeyondTheCombs.com

Made in United States
Orlando, FL
24 March 2023

31391058R00049